FAST FEAST DIET COOKBOOK FOR BEGINNERS

Revitalize Your Health with Nourishing Recipes for Rapid Results and Lasting Wellness.

ALASH MOHS

TABLE OF CONTENT

INTRODUCTION

Welcome to the Fast Feast Diet Cookbook, designed specifically for beginners who are eager to revitalize their health, achieve rapid results, and cultivate lasting wellness through nourishing and delicious recipes.

Whether you're new to the concept of intermittent fasting or looking to optimize your fasting routine, this cookbook is your comprehensive guide to embracing a healthier lifestyle without sacrificing flavor or satisfaction.

In recent years, intermittent fasting has gained immense popularity for its numerous health benefits, including weight loss, improved metabolic health, enhanced mental clarity, and longevity.

By strategically alternating between periods of eating and fasting, individuals can tap into their body's natural ability to burn fat, regulate blood sugar levels, and promote cellular repair and rejuvenation.

However, embarking on an intermittent fasting journey can feel daunting, especially for beginners who may be unsure of where to start or how to create balanced and nutritious meals within their fasting and feeding windows. That's where the Fast Feast Diet Cookbook comes in.

Inside these pages, you'll discover a diverse array of mouthwatering recipes that are not only delicious and satisfying but also perfectly aligned with the principles of intermittent fasting. From energizing breakfasts and hearty main courses to refreshing salads and indulgent desserts, each recipe has been thoughtfully crafted to support your health and well-being while keeping you on track with your fasting goals.

But this cookbook is more than just a collection of recipes—it's a comprehensive resource that will empower you to make informed choices about your diet and lifestyle. In addition to flavorful recipes, you'll find practical tips, expert advice, and valuable insights into the science behind intermittent fasting and its profound impact on your health.

Whether you're looking to shed excess weight, boost your energy levels, or simply improve your overall health and well-being, the Fast Feast Diet Cookbook is your ultimate companion on the journey to a healthier and happier you.

So, let's dive in and discover the transformative power of nourishing foods and intermittent fasting together.

Here's to a brighter, healthier future—one delicious meal at a time.

Quick and Easy Veggie Omelette

Ingredients:

- 2 eggs
- 1/4 cup bell peppers (any color), diced
- 1/4 cup onions, diced
- 1/4 cup spinach, chopped
- 1/4 cup tomatoes, diced
- 1/4 cup cheese (optional), shredded
- Salt and pepper to taste
- 1 tablespoon olive oil or butter for cooking

Instructions:

1. **Preparation:**
   - Crack the eggs into a mixing bowl and beat them until well combined.
   - Chop the bell peppers, onions, spinach, and tomatoes.
   - If using cheese, shred it and set it aside.

2. **Cooking:**

- Heat the olive oil or butter in a non-stick skillet over medium heat.

- Add the diced bell peppers and onions to the skillet and sauté for 2-3 minutes until they start to soften.

- Add the chopped spinach and tomatoes to the skillet and cook for another 1-2 minutes until the spinach wilts slightly.

3. **Making the Omelette:**

- Pour the beaten eggs over the sautéed vegetables in the skillet, ensuring that they spread out evenly.

- Allow the eggs to cook undisturbed for about 2-3 minutes until the edges start to set.

- Gently lift the edges of the omelette with a spatula and tilt the skillet to let the uncooked eggs flow to the edges.

- Sprinkle the shredded cheese (if using) evenly over one half of the omelette.

- Season the omelette with salt and pepper to taste.

4. **Finishing:**

- Once the eggs are almost set but still slightly runny on top, carefully fold the omelette in half using the spatula.

- Press down gently on the folded omelette with the spatula and cook for another 1-2 minutes until the cheese is melted and the omelette is cooked through.

5. **Serving:**

- Slide the cooked omelette onto a plate and serve hot.

- You can garnish the omelette with some extra chopped tomatoes, fresh herbs, or a dollop of salsa if desired.

Avocado Toast with Poached Egg

Ingredients:

- 1 ripe avocado
- 2 slices of whole grain bread
- 2 eggs
- Salt and pepper to taste
- Optional toppings: Red pepper flakes, chia seeds, sesame seeds, sliced cherry tomatoes, microgreens

Instructions:

1. **Prepare the Avocado:**

   - Cut the ripe avocado in half and remove the pit.
   - Scoop the avocado flesh into a bowl and mash it with a fork until smooth.
   - Season the mashed avocado with salt and pepper to taste.

2. **Toast the Bread:**

   - Toast the slices of whole grain bread until golden brown and crispy.

3. **Poach the Eggs:**

- Fill a medium-sized saucepan with water and bring it to a gentle simmer over medium heat.

- Crack one egg into a small bowl or ramekin.

- Using a spoon, create a gentle whirlpool in the simmering water and carefully slide the egg into the center of the whirlpool.

- Repeat the process with the second egg.

- Poach the eggs for about 3-4 minutes until the whites are set but the yolks are still runny.

- Use a slotted spoon to carefully remove the poached eggs from the water and transfer them to a plate lined with paper towels to drain any excess water.

4. **Assemble the Avocado Toast:**

- Spread a generous amount of mashed avocado onto each slice of toasted bread.

- Carefully place one poached egg on top of each avocado toast.

- Season the poached eggs with a sprinkle of salt and pepper.

5. **Optional Toppings:**

- Sprinkle the avocado toast with red pepper flakes, chia seeds, sesame seeds, or any other desired toppings for extra flavor and texture.

- Add sliced cherry tomatoes or microgreens for freshness and color.

6. **Serve and Enjoy:**

- Serve the Avocado Toast with Poached Egg immediately while still warm.

- Cut the toast in half or serve whole, depending on preference.

- Enjoy this delicious and nutritious breakfast or brunch option!

Recipe: Greek Yogurt Parfait

Ingredients:

- 1 cup Greek yogurt (plain or flavored)

- 1/2 cup mixed berries (strawberries, blueberries, raspberries)

- 2 tablespoons honey or maple syrup (optional)

- 1/4 cup granola or muesli

- Optional toppings: Sliced bananas, chopped nuts, shredded coconut, dark chocolate chips

Instructions:

1. **Prepare the Yogurt:**

   - If using plain Greek yogurt, you can sweeten it by stirring in honey or maple syrup to taste. Skip this step if using flavored Greek yogurt.

2. **Prepare the Berries:**

   - Wash the mixed berries thoroughly under cold water and pat them dry with a paper towel.

   - If using strawberries, hull and slice them into bite-sized pieces.

3. **Assemble the Parfait:**

- Start by spooning a layer of Greek yogurt into the bottom of a glass or serving dish.

- Add a layer of mixed berries on top of the yogurt.

- Sprinkle a layer of granola or muesli over the berries.

- Repeat the layers until you reach the top of the glass, finishing with a final layer of yogurt on top.

4. **Optional Toppings:**

- Garnish the Greek Yogurt Parfait with additional toppings of your choice, such as sliced bananas, chopped nuts, shredded coconut, or dark chocolate chips.

5. **Serve and Enjoy:**

- Serve the Greek Yogurt Parfait immediately, or cover and refrigerate it until ready to serve.

- Enjoy this delicious and nutritious parfait for breakfast, as a snack, or as a healthy dessert option!

Chia Seed Pudding

Ingredients:

- 1/4 cup chia seeds

- 1 cup almond milk (or any other milk of your choice)

- 1/2 teaspoon vanilla extract

- 1 tablespoon honey or maple syrup (optional)

- Fresh fruits (such as berries, sliced bananas, mango, or kiwi) for topping

- Nuts, seeds, or granola for topping (optional)

Instructions:

1. **Mix Chia Seeds and Milk:**

   - In a mixing bowl or glass jar, combine the chia seeds, almond milk, vanilla extract, and honey or maple syrup (if using).

   - Stir well to ensure that the chia seeds are evenly distributed in the milk mixture.

2. **Let it Set:**

- Once the ingredients are well combined, cover the bowl or jar and refrigerate the chia seed mixture for at least 4 hours or overnight.

- During this time, the chia seeds will absorb the liquid and swell up, creating a thick and pudding-like consistency.

3. **Stir and Serve:**

- After the chia seed pudding has set, remove it from the refrigerator and give it a good stir to break up any clumps.

- If the pudding is too thick for your liking, you can add a splash of almond milk to thin it out to your desired consistency.

4. **Assemble and Garnish:**

- Divide the chia seed pudding into serving bowls or jars.

- Top the pudding with your choice of fresh fruits, nuts, seeds, or granola for added flavor and texture.

5. **Serve and Enjoy:**

- Serve the Chia Seed Pudding immediately, or cover and store it in the refrigerator for up to 3-4 days.

- Enjoy this nutritious and delicious pudding for breakfast, as a snack, or as a healthy dessert option!

Quinoa Salad with Lemon Herb Dressing

Ingredients:

For the Salad:

- 1 cup quinoa, rinsed
- 2 cups water or vegetable broth
- 1 cucumber, diced
- 1 cup cherry tomatoes, halved
- 1/2 cup crumbled feta cheese
- 1/4 cup chopped fresh parsley
- Salt and pepper to taste

For the Lemon Herb Dressing:

- 1/4 cup extra virgin olive oil
- 2 tablespoons fresh lemon juice
- 1 teaspoon honey or maple syrup
- 1 teaspoon Dijon mustard
- 1 clove garlic, minced
- 1 tablespoon chopped fresh basil
- 1 tablespoon chopped fresh mint
- Salt and pepper to taste

Instructions:

1. **Cook the Quinoa:**

   - In a medium saucepan, combine the rinsed quinoa and water or vegetable broth.

   - Bring the mixture to a boil over medium-high heat.

   - Reduce the heat to low, cover, and simmer for 15-20 minutes, or until the quinoa is tender and the liquid is absorbed.

   - Remove the saucepan from the heat and let the quinoa cool to room temperature.

2. **Prepare the Salad Ingredients:**

   - While the quinoa is cooking, prepare the vegetables.

   - Dice the cucumber, halve the cherry tomatoes, and chop the fresh parsley.

3. **Make the Lemon Herb Dressing:**

   - In a small bowl, whisk together the extra virgin olive oil, fresh lemon juice, honey or maple syrup, Dijon mustard, minced garlic, chopped fresh basil, and chopped fresh mint.

- Season the dressing with salt and pepper to taste.

4. **Assemble the Salad:**

- In a large mixing bowl, combine the cooked quinoa, diced cucumber, halved cherry tomatoes, crumbled feta cheese, and chopped fresh parsley.

- Pour the lemon herb dressing over the salad ingredients and toss until everything is well coated.

- Taste and adjust the seasoning with salt and pepper if necessary.

5. **Serve and Enjoy:**

- Transfer the quinoa salad to a serving dish or individual bowls.

- Garnish with additional fresh herbs if desired.

- Serve the Quinoa Salad with Lemon Herb Dressing immediately, or cover and refrigerate until ready to serve.

- Enjoy this refreshing and flavorful salad as a light meal or side dish!

Zucchini Noodles with Pesto

Ingredients:

For the Zucchini Noodles:

- 4 medium zucchini
- Salt and pepper to taste

For the Pesto:

- 2 cups fresh basil leaves, packed
- 1/2 cup grated Parmesan cheese
- 1/2 cup pine nuts or walnuts
- 2 cloves garlic, peeled
- 1/2 cup extra virgin olive oil
- Salt and pepper to taste
- Optional: Lemon juice for extra flavor

Instructions:

1. **Prepare the Zucchini Noodles:**
   - Using a spiralizer or vegetable peeler, create zucchini noodles by shredding the zucchini lengthwise into thin strips.

- If using a spiralizer, follow the manufacturer's instructions for the desired noodle thickness.

- Place the zucchini noodles in a colander and sprinkle them with salt. Let them sit for about 10-15 minutes to release excess moisture.

- After the time has elapsed, gently squeeze the zucchini noodles to remove any remaining moisture. Set them aside.

2. **Make the Pesto:**

- In a food processor or blender, combine the fresh basil leaves, grated Parmesan cheese, pine nuts or walnuts, and peeled garlic cloves.

- Pulse the ingredients until they are finely chopped and well combined.

- While the food processor or blender is running, slowly drizzle in the extra virgin olive oil until the pesto reaches your desired consistency.

- Season the pesto with salt and pepper to taste, and optionally add a splash of lemon juice for extra flavor. Blend again to combine.

3. **Cook the Zucchini Noodles:**

- Heat a large skillet over medium heat and add a drizzle of olive oil.

- Once the skillet is hot, add the zucchini noodles and sauté them for 2-3 minutes, or until they are just tender but still slightly crisp.

- Season the zucchini noodles with salt and pepper to taste.

4. **Combine and Serve:**

- Transfer the cooked zucchini noodles to a serving dish.

- Spoon the freshly made pesto over the zucchini noodles and toss gently until they are evenly coated.

- Garnish with additional grated Parmesan cheese, pine nuts, or fresh basil leaves if desired.

- Serve the Zucchini Noodles with Pesto immediately as a light and flavorful meal or side dish.

Grilled Chicken Salad

Ingredients:

For the Grilled Chicken:

- 2 boneless, skinless chicken breasts
- 2 tablespoons olive oil
- 1 teaspoon garlic powder
- 1 teaspoon paprika
- Salt and pepper to taste

For the Salad:

- Mixed salad greens (such as lettuce, spinach, arugula)
- Cherry tomatoes, halved
- Cucumber, sliced
- Red onion, thinly sliced
- Avocado, sliced
- Optional toppings: Crumbled feta cheese, sliced almonds, dried cranberries

For the Dressing:

- 1/4 cup extra virgin olive oil
- 2 tablespoons balsamic vinegar

- 1 teaspoon Dijon mustard

- 1 teaspoon honey or maple syrup

- Salt and pepper to taste

Instructions:

1. **Prepare the Grilled Chicken:**

   - In a small bowl, mix together the olive oil, garlic powder, paprika, salt, and pepper to create a marinade.

   - Place the chicken breasts in a shallow dish or resealable plastic bag and pour the marinade over them, ensuring they are evenly coated.

   - Cover the dish or seal the bag and marinate the chicken in the refrigerator for at least 30 minutes, or up to 4 hours for maximum flavor.

   - Preheat the grill to medium-high heat.

   - Remove the chicken from the marinade and discard any excess marinade.

- Grill the chicken breasts for 6-8 minutes per side, or until they are cooked through and reach an internal temperature of 165°F (75°C).

- Remove the chicken from the grill and let it rest for a few minutes before slicing it thinly.

2. **Prepare the Salad Ingredients:**

- While the chicken is grilling, prepare the salad ingredients.

- Wash and dry the mixed salad greens, cherry tomatoes, cucumber, red onion, and avocado.

- Slice the cucumber, halve the cherry tomatoes, thinly slice the red onion, and slice the avocado.

3. **Make the Dressing:**

- In a small bowl or jar, whisk together the extra virgin olive oil, balsamic vinegar, Dijon mustard, honey or maple syrup, salt, and pepper until emulsified.

- Taste and adjust the seasoning if necessary.

4. **Assemble the Salad:**

- In a large salad bowl, combine the mixed salad greens, cherry tomatoes, cucumber, red onion, and avocado.

- Add the sliced grilled chicken on top of the salad.

5. **Serve:**

- Drizzle the balsamic vinaigrette dressing over the salad.

- Toss the salad gently until all ingredients are evenly coated with the dressing.

- Optional: Sprinkle crumbled feta cheese, sliced almonds, or dried cranberries on top for extra flavor and texture.

- Serve the Grilled Chicken Salad immediately as a satisfying and nutritious meal.

Salmon with Asparagus

Ingredients:

For the Salmon:

- 2 salmon fillets
- 2 tablespoons olive oil
- 2 cloves garlic, minced
- 1 lemon, sliced
- Salt and pepper to taste

For the Asparagus:

- 1 bunch asparagus, trimmed
- 1 tablespoon olive oil
- Salt and pepper to taste

Instructions:

1. **Preheat the Oven:**
   - Preheat your oven to 400°F (200°C).

2. **Prepare the Salmon:**
   - Place the salmon fillets on a baking sheet lined with parchment paper or aluminum foil.

- Drizzle olive oil over the salmon fillets and rub minced garlic onto them.

- Season the salmon fillets generously with salt and pepper.

- Place lemon slices on top of each salmon fillet.

3. **Prepare the Asparagus:**

- Trim the tough ends off the asparagus spears.

- Place the asparagus on the same baking sheet as the salmon.

- Drizzle olive oil over the asparagus and toss to coat evenly.

- Season the asparagus with salt and pepper.

4. **Bake the Salmon and Asparagus:**

- Transfer the baking sheet to the preheated oven and bake for 12-15 minutes, or until the salmon is cooked through and flakes easily with a fork.

- The cooking time may vary depending on the thickness of the salmon fillets, so adjust accordingly.

5. **Serve:**

- Once the salmon and asparagus are cooked, remove them from the oven.

- Carefully transfer the salmon fillets and asparagus to serving plates.

- Serve the Salmon with Asparagus hot, garnished with additional lemon slices if desired.

- Enjoy this delicious and nutritious meal!

Turkey Lettuce Wraps

Ingredients:

For the Turkey Filling:

- 1 lb ground turkey
- 2 tablespoons olive oil
- 1 small onion, diced
- 2 cloves garlic, minced
- 1 red bell pepper, diced
- 1 tablespoon soy sauce
- 1 teaspoon ground ginger
- Salt and pepper to taste
- Butter lettuce leaves, for wrapping

For the Topping (Optional):

- Sliced green onions
- Chopped cilantro
- Sliced radishes
- Sliced cucumber
- Sriracha or chili sauce

Instructions:

1. **Cook the Turkey Filling:**

- Heat olive oil in a large skillet over medium heat.

- Add diced onion and minced garlic to the skillet and cook until softened and fragrant, about 2-3 minutes.

- Add ground turkey to the skillet and cook, breaking it up with a spatula, until browned and cooked through.

- Stir in diced red bell pepper, soy sauce, and ground ginger. Cook for another 2-3 minutes until the bell pepper is tender.

- Season the turkey filling with salt and pepper to taste.

2. **Prepare the Lettuce Wraps:**

- Rinse and dry the butter lettuce leaves, then lay them out flat on a serving platter.

- Spoon the cooked turkey filling onto each lettuce leaf, dividing it evenly among them.

3. **Add Toppings (Optional):**

- Garnish the turkey lettuce wraps with sliced green onions, chopped cilantro, sliced radishes, sliced cucumber, or any other desired toppings.

- Drizzle with sriracha or chili sauce for added flavor and heat, if desired.

4. **Serve:**

- Serve the Turkey Lettuce Wraps immediately, allowing everyone to assemble their own wraps at the table.

- Enjoy these flavorful and satisfying lettuce wraps as a healthy and delicious meal or appetizer!

Vegetable Stir-Fry

Ingredients:

For the Stir-Fry:

- 2 tablespoons vegetable oil
- 2 cloves garlic, minced
- 1-inch piece of ginger, minced
- 1 onion, thinly sliced
- 2 bell peppers (any color), thinly sliced
- 2 cups broccoli florets
- 1 cup snap peas, trimmed
- 2 carrots, julienned
- 1 cup mushrooms, sliced
- 1 cup tofu or chicken, cubed (optional)
- Salt and pepper to taste

For the Sauce:

- 1/4 cup soy sauce
- 2 tablespoons oyster sauce
- 1 tablespoon rice vinegar
- 1 tablespoon honey or maple syrup
- 1 teaspoon sesame oil

- 1 teaspoon cornstarch (optional, for thickening)

Optional Garnishes:

- Sliced green onions

- Sesame seeds

- Crushed red pepper flakes

Instructions:

1. **Prepare the Sauce:**

   - In a small bowl, whisk together soy sauce, oyster sauce, rice vinegar, honey or maple syrup, sesame oil, and cornstarch (if using). Set aside.

2. **Cook the Protein (Optional):**

   - If using tofu or chicken, heat 1 tablespoon of vegetable oil in a large skillet or wok over medium-high heat.

   - Add the cubed tofu or chicken to the skillet and cook until browned and cooked through. Remove from the skillet and set aside.

3. **Stir-Fry the Vegetables:**

- Heat the remaining tablespoon of vegetable oil in the same skillet or wok over medium-high heat.

- Add minced garlic and ginger to the skillet and cook for 1 minute until fragrant.

- Add sliced onion to the skillet and cook for 2-3 minutes until softened.

- Add sliced bell peppers, broccoli florets, snap peas, julienned carrots, and sliced mushrooms to the skillet. Cook for 5-6 minutes, stirring frequently, until the vegetables are tender-crisp.

4. **Combine and Cook:**

- Return the cooked protein (if using) to the skillet with the vegetables.

- Pour the prepared sauce over the stir-fry mixture in the skillet.

- Stir well to coat everything evenly in the sauce.

- Cook for an additional 2-3 minutes, or until the sauce has thickened slightly and everything is heated through.

- Season with salt and pepper to taste.

5. **Serve:**

    - Transfer the Vegetable Stir-Fry to a serving dish or individual plates.

    - Garnish with sliced green onions, sesame seeds, or crushed red pepper flakes if desired.

    - Serve the stir-fry hot over cooked rice or noodles, or enjoy it on its own as a healthy and flavorful meal!

Mango and Black Bean Salad

Ingredients:

- 1 ripe mango, peeled and diced
- 1 can (15 ounces) black beans, rinsed and drained
- 1 red bell pepper, diced
- 1/2 red onion, finely chopped
- 1 jalapeño pepper, seeded and finely chopped (optional)
- 1/4 cup fresh cilantro, chopped
- Juice of 2 limes
- 2 tablespoons olive oil
- Salt and pepper to taste
- Optional: Avocado slices for garnish

Instructions:

1. **Prepare the Ingredients:**
   - Peel and dice the ripe mango.
   - Rinse and drain the black beans.
   - Dice the red bell pepper.
   - Finely chop the red onion.

- Seed and finely chop the jalapeño pepper if using.

- Chop the fresh cilantro.

2. Combine the Ingredients:

- In a large mixing bowl, combine the diced mango, black beans, diced red bell pepper, finely chopped red onion, chopped jalapeño pepper (if using), and chopped cilantro.

3. Make the Dressing:

- In a small bowl, whisk together the lime juice and olive oil until well combined.

- Season the dressing with salt and pepper to taste.

4. Toss the Salad:

- Pour the dressing over the mango and black bean mixture in the large mixing bowl.

- Gently toss the salad until all ingredients are evenly coated with the dressing.

5. Chill (Optional):

- If time allows, cover the salad and refrigerate it for at least 30 minutes to allow the flavors to meld together.

6. **Serve:**

   - Once chilled (if desired), transfer the Mango and Black Bean Salad to a serving dish.

   - Garnish with avocado slices if using.

   - Serve the salad as a refreshing side dish or as a light and healthy meal on its own.

   - Enjoy!

Caprese Salad

Ingredients:

- 2 large ripe tomatoes, sliced
- 1 ball fresh mozzarella cheese, sliced
- Fresh basil leaves
- Extra virgin olive oil
- Balsamic glaze (or balsamic vinegar)
- Salt and pepper to taste

Instructions:

1. **Prepare the Ingredients:**

   - Wash and dry the tomatoes and basil leaves.
   - Slice the tomatoes and fresh mozzarella cheese into uniform slices.

2. **Assemble the Salad:**

   - Arrange the tomato slices on a serving platter or individual plates.
   - Place a slice of fresh mozzarella cheese on top of each tomato slice.
   - Tuck fresh basil leaves in between the tomato and mozzarella slices.

3. **Drizzle with Olive Oil:**

   - Drizzle extra virgin olive oil over the tomato, mozzarella, and basil slices.

   - Use a light hand to avoid over-saturating the salad.

4. **Season with Salt and Pepper:**

   - Sprinkle salt and pepper over the Caprese salad to taste.

   - Remember that the mozzarella cheese may already contain some salt, so adjust accordingly.

5. **Finish with Balsamic Glaze:**

   - Drizzle balsamic glaze (or balsamic vinegar) over the Caprese salad for added flavor and presentation.

   - If using balsamic glaze, drizzle it in a zig-zag pattern over the salad.

   - If using balsamic vinegar, you can either drizzle it directly over the salad or serve it on the side for individual preference.

6. **Serve:**

- Serve the Caprese Salad immediately as a refreshing appetizer or side dish.

- Enjoy the combination of ripe tomatoes, creamy mozzarella, and fragrant basil, enhanced by the richness of extra virgin olive oil and the sweetness of balsamic glaze.

Eggplant and Chickpea Curry

Ingredients:

- 1 large eggplant, diced
- 1 can (15 ounces) chickpeas, rinsed and drained
- 1 onion, diced
- 2 cloves garlic, minced
- 1 tablespoon fresh ginger, grated
- 1 can (14 ounces) diced tomatoes
- 1 can (14 ounces) coconut milk
- 1 tablespoon curry powder
- 1 teaspoon ground cumin
- 1 teaspoon ground coriander
- 1/2 teaspoon turmeric powder
- 1/4 teaspoon cayenne pepper (optional, for heat)
- Salt and pepper to taste
- Fresh cilantro, chopped (for garnish)
- Cooked rice or naan bread, for serving

Instructions:

1. **Prepare the Ingredients:**

   - Wash and dice the eggplant into bite-sized pieces.

   - Rinse and drain the chickpeas.

   - Dice the onion, mince the garlic, and grate the fresh ginger.

2. **Cook the Aromatics:**

   - Heat a large skillet or pot over medium heat.

   - Add a splash of oil to the skillet and add the diced onion.

   - Cook the onion for 2-3 minutes until it begins to soften.

   - Add the minced garlic and grated ginger to the skillet and cook for an additional minute until fragrant.

3. **Add the Spices:**

   - Sprinkle the curry powder, ground cumin, ground coriander, turmeric powder, and cayenne pepper (if using) over the cooked aromatics.

   - Stir well to toast the spices for 1-2 minutes until fragrant.

4. **Cook the Eggplant and Chickpeas:**

- Add the diced eggplant and rinsed chickpeas to the skillet.

- Stir to coat the eggplant and chickpeas with the spices and aromatics.

5. **Add the Tomatoes and Coconut Milk:**

- Pour the diced tomatoes and coconut milk into the skillet with the eggplant and chickpeas.

- Stir well to combine all the ingredients.

6. **Simmer the Curry:**

- Bring the mixture to a gentle simmer, then reduce the heat to low.

- Cover the skillet and let the curry simmer for 15-20 minutes, stirring occasionally, until the eggplant is tender and the flavors have melded together.

7. **Season and Serve:**

- Taste the curry and season with salt and pepper to taste.

- If the curry is too thick, you can add a splash of water to thin it out.

- Garnish the Eggplant and Chickpea Curry with freshly chopped cilantro.

- Serve the curry hot over cooked rice or with naan bread on the side.

Shrimp and Veggie Skewers

Ingredients:

- 1 lb large shrimp, peeled and deveined
- 1 red bell pepper, cut into chunks
- 1 yellow bell pepper, cut into chunks
- 1 zucchini, sliced into rounds
- 1 red onion, cut into chunks
- 1 lemon, sliced (optional, for garnish)
- Wooden or metal skewers, soaked if using wooden skewers
- Salt and pepper to taste
- Olive oil for brushing

Instructions:

1. **Prepare the Shrimp:**

   - If using wooden skewers, soak them in water for at least 30 minutes to prevent them from burning.
   - Peel and devein the shrimp if they haven't been already.

- Pat the shrimp dry with paper towels and season with salt and pepper to taste.

2. **Prepare the Vegetables:**

   - Wash and chop the red and yellow bell peppers into chunks.

   - Slice the zucchini into rounds.

   - Cut the red onion into chunks.

3. **Assemble the Skewers:**

   - Thread the shrimp, bell peppers, zucchini slices, and red onion chunks onto the skewers, alternating between the ingredients.

   - Leave a little space between each ingredient to ensure even cooking.

   - Repeat until all ingredients are used up.

4. **Brush with Olive Oil:**

   - Preheat the grill to medium-high heat.

   - Brush the assembled skewers with olive oil to prevent sticking and promote even grilling.

5. **Grill the Skewers:**

- Place the skewers on the preheated grill and cook for 2-3 minutes per side, or until the shrimp are pink and opaque and the vegetables are tender and slightly charred.

- If using wooden skewers, be sure to rotate them occasionally to ensure even cooking.

6. **Serve:**

- Once cooked, remove the skewers from the grill and transfer them to a serving platter.

- Garnish with lemon slices if desired.

- Serve the Shrimp and Veggie Skewers hot as a delicious and nutritious main course or appetizer.

Mushroom and Spinach Quesadillas

Ingredients:

- 8 large flour tortillas

- 2 cups sliced mushrooms (such as button or cremini)

- 2 cups fresh spinach leaves

- 1 small onion, finely chopped

- 2 cloves garlic, minced

- 1 cup shredded Monterey Jack cheese

- 1 cup shredded cheddar cheese

- 2 tablespoons olive oil

- Salt and pepper to taste

- Optional toppings: Sliced avocado, sour cream, salsa

Instructions:

1. **Prepare the Filling:**

   - Heat 1 tablespoon of olive oil in a large skillet over medium heat.

   - Add the sliced mushrooms to the skillet and cook for 5-6 minutes, stirring occasionally, until they are browned and tender.

- Remove the mushrooms from the skillet and set aside.

- In the same skillet, add the remaining tablespoon of olive oil.

- Add the chopped onion to the skillet and cook for 2-3 minutes until softened.

- Add the minced garlic to the skillet and cook for an additional minute until fragrant.

- Add the fresh spinach leaves to the skillet and cook for 1-2 minutes until wilted.

- Season the mushroom and spinach mixture with salt and pepper to taste.

- Remove the skillet from the heat and set aside.

2. **Assemble the Quesadillas:**

- Lay out 4 flour tortillas on a flat surface.

- Divide the shredded Monterey Jack and cheddar cheese evenly among the tortillas, spreading it out in an even layer.

- Spoon the cooked mushroom and spinach mixture evenly over the cheese layer.

- Top each quesadilla with another flour tortilla to form a sandwich.

3. **Cook the Quesadillas:**

- Heat a large skillet or griddle over medium heat.

- Place one of the assembled quesadillas in the skillet and cook for 2-3 minutes on each side, or until the tortilla is golden brown and the cheese is melted.

- Repeat with the remaining quesadillas, cooking them in batches if necessary.

4. **Serve:**

- Once cooked, remove the quesadillas from the skillet and transfer them to a cutting board.

- Use a sharp knife to cut each quesadilla into wedges.

- Serve the Mushroom and Spinach Quesadillas hot with optional toppings such as sliced avocado, sour cream, or salsa.

- Enjoy this delicious and satisfying meal!

Sweet Potato and Black Bean Tacos

Ingredients:

- 2 large sweet potatoes, peeled and diced
- 1 can (15 ounces) black beans, rinsed and drained
- 1 red bell pepper, diced
- 1 small red onion, diced
- 2 cloves garlic, minced
- 1 teaspoon chili powder
- 1/2 teaspoon ground cumin
- 1/2 teaspoon smoked paprika
- Salt and pepper to taste
- 8 small flour or corn tortillas
- Toppings:
  - Avocado slices
  - Salsa
  - Shredded lettuce
  - Fresh cilantro
  - Lime wedges

Instructions:

1. **Prepare the Sweet Potatoes:**

   - Peel the sweet potatoes and dice them into small cubes.

2. **Cook the Sweet Potatoes:**

   - Heat a large skillet over medium heat and add a drizzle of olive oil.

   - Add the diced sweet potatoes to the skillet and cook for 8-10 minutes, stirring occasionally, until they are tender and lightly browned.

   - Add the minced garlic to the skillet and cook for an additional minute until fragrant.

3. **Prepare the Black Bean Mixture:**

   - Add the rinsed and drained black beans, diced red bell pepper, and diced red onion to the skillet with the cooked sweet potatoes.

   - Season the mixture with chili powder, ground cumin, smoked paprika, salt, and pepper.

   - Stir well to combine all ingredients.

- Cook for another 3-4 minutes until the black bean mixture is heated through and the flavors have melded together.

4. **Warm the Tortillas:**

   - While the sweet potato and black bean mixture is cooking, warm the tortillas.

   - Heat a dry skillet over medium heat and warm each tortilla for about 30 seconds on each side until softened and heated through.

   - Alternatively, you can wrap the tortillas in damp paper towels and microwave them for 30-60 seconds until warmed.

5. **Assemble the Tacos:**

   - Spoon the sweet potato and black bean mixture onto each warmed tortilla.

   - Top with avocado slices, salsa, shredded lettuce, fresh cilantro, and a squeeze of lime juice.

   - Feel free to customize the toppings according to your preference.

6. **Serve:**

- Serve the Sweet Potato and Black Bean Tacos immediately, garnished with additional cilantro and lime wedges if desired.

- Enjoy these flavorful and satisfying tacos as a delicious meatless meal option!

Cauliflower Fried Rice

Ingredients:

- 1 medium head of cauliflower
- 2 tablespoons sesame oil
- 2 cloves garlic, minced
- 1 small onion, diced
- 1 cup mixed vegetables (such as carrots, peas, and corn)
- 2 eggs, beaten
- 3 tablespoons soy sauce
- 1 teaspoon sriracha sauce (optional, for heat)
- Salt and pepper to taste
- Green onions, chopped (for garnish)
- Sesame seeds (for garnish)

Instructions:

1. **Prepare the Cauliflower Rice:**
   - Remove the leaves and core from the cauliflower head.
   - Cut the cauliflower into florets and place them in a food processor.

- Pulse the cauliflower florets in the food processor until they resemble rice or couscous-sized grains. Be careful not to overprocess.

2. **Cook the Cauliflower Rice:**

   - Heat 1 tablespoon of sesame oil in a large skillet or wok over medium heat.

   - Add the minced garlic and diced onion to the skillet and cook for 2-3 minutes until softened and fragrant.

   - Add the riced cauliflower and mixed vegetables to the skillet.

   - Stir-fry the cauliflower and vegetables for 5-6 minutes, stirring occasionally, until the cauliflower is tender but still slightly crisp.

   - Season with salt and pepper to taste.

3. **Scramble the Eggs:**

   - Push the cauliflower mixture to one side of the skillet to create a clear space.

- Pour the beaten eggs into the clear space and let them cook for a few seconds until they start to set.

- Use a spatula to scramble the eggs, breaking them into small pieces as they cook.

4. **Combine and Season:**

   - Once the eggs are cooked, stir them into the cauliflower mixture until evenly distributed.

   - Drizzle the remaining tablespoon of sesame oil over the fried rice.

   - Add soy sauce and sriracha sauce (if using) to the skillet and toss everything together until well combined.

   - Taste and adjust the seasoning with salt and pepper if necessary.

5. **Garnish and Serve:**

   - Remove the skillet from the heat and transfer the Cauliflower Fried Rice to a serving dish.

   - Garnish with chopped green onions and sesame seeds for added flavor and presentation.

- Serve the fried rice hot as a delicious and healthy alternative to traditional rice-based dishes.

Stuffed Bell Peppers

Ingredients:

- 4 large bell peppers (any color)
- 1 lb ground beef or turkey
- 1 cup cooked rice (white or brown)
- 1 small onion, diced
- 2 cloves garlic, minced
- 1 can (14 ounces) diced tomatoes, drained
- 1 cup shredded cheese (such as cheddar or mozzarella)
- 1 teaspoon dried oregano
- 1 teaspoon dried basil
- Salt and pepper to taste
- Olive oil for cooking
- Optional toppings: Chopped fresh parsley, sliced green onions, sour cream, salsa

Instructions:

1. **Prepare the Bell Peppers:**
   - Preheat your oven to 375°F (190°C).

- Cut the tops off the bell peppers and remove the seeds and membranes from inside.

- If necessary, slice a small portion off the bottom of each pepper to create a flat surface for them to stand upright in the baking dish.

2. **Cook the Filling:**

- Heat a tablespoon of olive oil in a large skillet over medium heat.

- Add the diced onion and minced garlic to the skillet and cook for 2-3 minutes until softened and fragrant.

- Add the ground beef or turkey to the skillet and cook, breaking it up with a spatula, until browned and cooked through.

- Drain any excess fat from the skillet.

- Stir in the cooked rice, drained diced tomatoes, dried oregano, dried basil, salt, and pepper. Cook for an additional 2-3 minutes until heated through and well combined.

3. **Stuff the Bell Peppers:**

- Place the hollowed-out bell peppers upright in a baking dish.

- Spoon the filling mixture into each bell pepper until they are full.

- Press down gently to pack the filling into the peppers.

4. **Bake the Stuffed Bell Peppers:**

- Sprinkle shredded cheese over the tops of the stuffed bell peppers.

- Cover the baking dish with aluminum foil and bake in the preheated oven for 25-30 minutes.

5. **Serve:**

- Once the stuffed bell peppers are cooked through and the cheese is melted and bubbly, remove them from the oven.

- Garnish with chopped fresh parsley or sliced green onions if desired.

- Serve the Stuffed Bell Peppers hot with optional toppings such as sour cream or salsa.

- Enjoy this hearty and satisfying meal!

Tuna Salad Lettuce Wraps

Ingredients:

- 2 cans (5 ounces each) tuna in water, drained

- 1/4 cup mayonnaise

- 1 tablespoon Dijon mustard

- 1 tablespoon lemon juice

- 1/4 cup diced celery

- 1/4 cup diced red onion

- 2 tablespoons chopped fresh parsley

- Salt and pepper to taste

- Butter lettuce leaves, washed and dried

- Optional toppings: Sliced avocado, cherry tomatoes, cucumber slices

Instructions:

1. **Prepare the Tuna Salad:**

   - In a medium-sized mixing bowl, combine the drained tuna, mayonnaise, Dijon mustard, lemon juice, diced celery, diced red onion, and chopped fresh parsley.

- Stir the ingredients together until well combined.

- Season the tuna salad with salt and pepper to taste. Adjust seasoning as needed.

2. **Assemble the Lettuce Wraps:**

- Lay out the butter lettuce leaves on a clean surface.

- Spoon a generous portion of the tuna salad onto each lettuce leaf, spreading it out evenly.

3. **Add Optional Toppings:**

- If desired, top each tuna salad-filled lettuce wrap with sliced avocado, halved cherry tomatoes, or cucumber slices for added flavor and texture.

4. **Wrap and Serve:**

- Carefully fold the sides of each lettuce leaf over the tuna salad filling.

- Roll up the lettuce leaves from the bottom to form tight wraps.

- Secure the wraps with toothpicks if necessary to hold them together.

- Serve the Tuna Salad Lettuce Wraps immediately as a light and refreshing meal or snack.

- Enjoy the delicious combination of creamy tuna salad wrapped in crisp, fresh lettuce leaves!

Mediterranean Couscous Salad

Ingredients:

- 1 cup couscous
- 1 1/4 cups vegetable broth or water
- 1 cup cherry tomatoes, halved
- 1 cucumber, diced
- 1/2 red onion, finely chopped
- 1/4 cup Kalamata olives, pitted and sliced
- 1/4 cup crumbled feta cheese
- 2 tablespoons chopped fresh parsley
- 2 tablespoons chopped fresh mint
- 2 tablespoons extra virgin olive oil
- 2 tablespoons lemon juice
- 1 clove garlic, minced
- Salt and pepper to taste

Instructions:

1. **Cook the Couscous:**

   - In a medium saucepan, bring the vegetable broth or water to a boil.

- Stir in the couscous, cover the saucepan, and remove it from the heat.

- Let the couscous steam for 5 minutes.

- Fluff the couscous with a fork to separate the grains.

2. **Prepare the Dressing:**

   - In a small bowl, whisk together the extra virgin olive oil, lemon juice, minced garlic, salt, and pepper to make the dressing.

3. **Assemble the Salad:**

   - In a large mixing bowl, combine the cooked couscous, halved cherry tomatoes, diced cucumber, finely chopped red onion, sliced Kalamata olives, crumbled feta cheese, chopped fresh parsley, and chopped fresh mint.

4. **Add the Dressing:**

   - Pour the prepared dressing over the couscous salad ingredients in the mixing bowl.

- Toss everything together until well combined and evenly coated with the dressing.

5. **Chill (Optional):**

   - Cover the bowl and refrigerate the Mediterranean Couscous Salad for at least 30 minutes to allow the flavors to meld together.

6. **Serve:**

   - Once chilled (if desired), transfer the couscous salad to a serving dish or individual plates.

   - Garnish with additional chopped fresh parsley and mint if desired.

   - Serve the Mediterranean Couscous Salad as a delicious and refreshing side dish or light meal.

   - Enjoy the vibrant flavors of the Mediterranean in every bite!

Hummus and Veggie Wrap

Ingredients:

- 1 large whole wheat or spinach tortilla

- 2 tablespoons hummus (store-bought or homemade)

- 1/4 cup shredded carrots

- 1/4 cup sliced cucumber

- 1/4 cup sliced bell peppers (any color)

- 1/4 cup baby spinach leaves

- 2 tablespoons crumbled feta cheese (optional)

- Salt and pepper to taste

Instructions:

1. **Prepare the Tortilla:**

    - Lay the whole wheat or spinach tortilla flat on a clean surface.

2. **Spread the Hummus:**

    - Spread the hummus evenly over the surface of the tortilla, leaving a small border around the edges.

3. **Layer the Veggies:**

- Arrange the shredded carrots, sliced cucumber, sliced bell peppers, and baby spinach leaves in a single layer on top of the hummus-covered tortilla.

- If using crumbled feta cheese, sprinkle it evenly over the veggies.

4. **Season with Salt and Pepper:**

   - Season the veggies with a sprinkle of salt and pepper to taste, if desired.

5. **Roll the Wrap:**

   - Starting from one end of the tortilla, tightly roll it up into a wrap, enclosing the hummus and veggies inside.

   - Tuck in the sides of the tortilla as you roll to prevent the filling from spilling out.

6. **Slice and Serve:**

   - Once rolled, use a sharp knife to slice the Hummus and Veggie Wrap in half or into smaller pinwheels.

   - Serve immediately, or wrap the halves or pinwheels in parchment paper or foil for easy transport and enjoy on the go!

Optional: You can also toast the wrap in a panini press or on a skillet for a warm and crispy variation.

Turkey and Veggie Lettuce Wraps

Ingredients:

- 1 lb ground turkey
- 1 tablespoon olive oil
- 2 cloves garlic, minced
- 1 small onion, diced
- 1 bell pepper (any color), diced
- 1 cup shredded carrots
- 1 cup shredded cabbage
- 1/4 cup hoisin sauce
- 2 tablespoons soy sauce
- 1 tablespoon rice vinegar
- 1 teaspoon sesame oil
- 1 teaspoon grated fresh ginger
- Salt and pepper to taste
- Butter lettuce leaves, washed and dried

Instructions:

1. **Cook the Turkey:**

- Heat olive oil in a large skillet over medium heat.

- Add minced garlic and diced onion to the skillet and cook for 2-3 minutes until softened and fragrant.

- Add ground turkey to the skillet and cook, breaking it up with a spatula, until browned and cooked through.

2. **Add the Veggies:**

   - Stir in diced bell pepper, shredded carrots, and shredded cabbage to the skillet with the cooked turkey.

   - Cook for an additional 3-4 minutes until the vegetables are tender-crisp.

3. **Make the Sauce:**

   - In a small bowl, whisk together hoisin sauce, soy sauce, rice vinegar, sesame oil, and grated fresh ginger until well combined.

   - Pour the sauce over the turkey and veggie mixture in the skillet.

   - Stir well to coat everything evenly in the sauce.

- Cook for another 1-2 minutes until heated through.

- Season with salt and pepper to taste.

4. **Assemble the Lettuce Wraps:**

- Spoon the turkey and veggie mixture onto individual butter lettuce leaves.

- Roll up the lettuce leaves around the filling, forming tight wraps.

- Secure the wraps with toothpicks if necessary to hold them together.

5. **Serve:**

- Arrange the Turkey and Veggie Lettuce Wraps on a serving platter.

- Serve immediately as a healthy and flavorful meal or appetizer.

- Enjoy the delicious combination of tender turkey and crunchy vegetables wrapped in crisp lettuce leaves!

Fruit Salad with Honey-Lime Dressing

Ingredients:

For the Fruit Salad:

- 2 cups strawberries, hulled and sliced
- 1 cup blueberries
- 1 cup grapes, halved
- 2 kiwis, peeled and sliced
- 1 mango, peeled and diced
- 1 banana, sliced
- 1 orange, peeled and segmented
- 1 apple, diced
- 1 cup pineapple chunks

For the Honey-Lime Dressing:

- 3 tablespoons honey
- 2 tablespoons freshly squeezed lime juice
- 1 teaspoon lime zest
- 1 tablespoon chopped fresh mint leaves (optional)

Instructions:

1. **Prepare the Fruit:**

   - Wash, hull, peel, and slice all the fruits as needed according to the ingredient list.

2. **Combine the Fruits:**

   - In a large mixing bowl, combine all the prepared fruits: strawberries, blueberries, grapes, kiwis, mango, banana, orange segments, apple, and pineapple chunks.

   - Gently toss the fruits together to mix them evenly.

3. **Make the Honey-Lime Dressing:**

   - In a small bowl, whisk together honey, lime juice, and lime zest until well combined.

   - Optionally, stir in chopped fresh mint leaves for extra flavor.

4. **Dress the Fruit Salad:**

   - Drizzle the prepared Honey-Lime Dressing over the mixed fruits in the large bowl.

5. **Toss and Chill:**

- Gently toss the fruits with the dressing until evenly coated.

- Cover the bowl and refrigerate the fruit salad for at least 30 minutes to allow the flavors to meld together and the salad to chill.

6. **Serve:**

- Once chilled, give the fruit salad a final toss.

- Transfer the fruit salad to a serving bowl or individual dishes.

- Optionally, garnish with additional fresh mint leaves or lime zest for presentation.

- Serve the Fruit Salad with Honey-Lime Dressing as a refreshing and nutritious dessert or side dish.

- Enjoy the vibrant flavors and colors of the mixed fruits combined with the sweet and tangy dressing!

Chicken and Vegetable Skillet

Ingredients:

- 1 lb boneless, skinless chicken breasts, cut into bite-sized pieces

- 2 tablespoons olive oil

- 1 onion, diced

- 2 cloves garlic, minced

- 1 bell pepper (any color), diced

- 1 zucchini, diced

- 1 cup cherry tomatoes, halved

- 2 cups baby spinach leaves

- 1 teaspoon dried oregano

- 1 teaspoon dried thyme

- Salt and pepper to taste

- Grated Parmesan cheese for garnish (optional)

Instructions:

1. **Cook the Chicken:**

   - Heat olive oil in a large skillet over medium-high heat.

- Add the diced chicken pieces to the skillet and cook for 5-6 minutes, stirring occasionally, until browned and cooked through.

- Once cooked, remove the chicken from the skillet and set it aside.

2. **Cook the Vegetables:**

   - In the same skillet, add a little more olive oil if needed.

   - Add diced onion and minced garlic to the skillet and cook for 2-3 minutes until softened and fragrant.

   - Add diced bell pepper and zucchini to the skillet and cook for an additional 4-5 minutes until they start to soften.

   - Stir in halved cherry tomatoes, dried oregano, and dried thyme. Cook for another 2 minutes until the tomatoes start to soften.

3. **Combine Chicken and Vegetables:**

   - Return the cooked chicken to the skillet with the vegetables.

   - Add baby spinach leaves to the skillet and stir everything together.

- Cook for an additional 1-2 minutes until the spinach wilts and the chicken is heated through.

- Season with salt and pepper to taste.

4. **Serve:**

- Once everything is cooked through and well combined, remove the skillet from the heat.

- Optionally, sprinkle grated Parmesan cheese over the chicken and vegetable skillet for added flavor.

- Serve the Chicken and Vegetable Skillet hot as a delicious and nutritious meal.

- Enjoy the flavorful combination of tender chicken and colorful vegetables in every bite!

CONCLUSION

As we reach the end of the Fast Feast Diet Cookbook for beginners, it's important to reflect on the transformative journey we've embarked upon together.

Through the pages of this cookbook, we've explored the powerful synergy between nourishing recipes and intermittent fasting, discovering how these two elements can work in harmony to revitalize our health, achieve rapid results, and foster lasting wellness.

We've learned that intermittent fasting is not just a diet, but a lifestyle approach that harnesses the body's innate ability to heal, regenerate, and thrive.

By strategically incorporating periods of fasting and feeding into our routine, we've unlocked a multitude of health benefits—from weight loss and improved metabolic health to increased energy levels and mental clarity.

But perhaps most importantly, we've discovered that nourishing our bodies with wholesome, nutrient-rich foods is the cornerstone of any successful fasting regimen.

The recipes in this cookbook have been carefully curated to provide a balance of essential nutrients, flavors, and textures, ensuring that every meal is not only delicious and satisfying but also supports our health and well-being.

As we conclude our journey with the Fast Feast Diet Cookbook, let us carry forward the valuable lessons and insights we've gained into our daily lives.

Let us continue to nourish our bodies with wholesome foods, embrace the practice of intermittent fasting as a tool for optimal health, and cultivate a mindset of mindfulness and balance in all aspects of our lives.

Remember, the path to lasting wellness is not a destination, but a continuous journey of self-discovery, growth, and transformation. And with the knowledge and recipes contained within these pages, you have everything you need to embark on that journey with confidence, determination, and joy.

Here's to your health, vitality, and happiness—may your future be filled with abundant blessings and delicious meals that nourish both body and soul.

Bon appétit, and cheers to your health and wellness journey!

With Warmest Wishes!!